T0209387

MY FAMILY
BOOK OF WORKOUTS AND
INSPIRATIONAL QUOTES

Great Lessons for the **Body, Mind and Soul**

FREDDIE MANGANO

BALBOA.PRESS

A DIVISION OF HAY HOUSE

Balboa Press books may be ordered through booksellers or by contacting:

Balboa Press
A Division of Hay House
1663 Liberty Drive
Bloomington, IN 47403
www.balboapress.com
1 (877) 407-4847

Print information available on the last page.

ISBN: 978-1-9822-4758-4 (sc)
ISBN: 978-1-9822-4760-7 (hc)
ISBN: 978-1-9822-4759-1 (e)

Library of Congress Control Number: 2020909238

Balboa Press rev. date: 05/28/2020

DEDICATION

I dedicate this book to my beloved brother David, and my loving father "Big" John, who have gone ahead to Heaven without me for now. But, I have a feeling they are still working out together in a huge, beautiful gym in the sky!

CONTENTS

ACKNOWLEDGEMENTS

This book would have not have been possible without the love and support of my Beautiful wife, Maria. She has always been in my corner with every venture I undertake. She is my rock. Words cannot express my gratitude for her. Also, our son Joseph, actually, Joseph is my stepson who I say, if I had to order a child, he would be the one. So thank you LORD for Joseph, who also backs me up in all I do in this life.

To my Family, who, through the many years of crazy ideas have never failed to believe in me. My mom Rita is always there to support me from when I was ten years old and thinking about becoming an actor to when I went into business with my brother David. David also was one of my biggest supporters of any business we went into, either together, or as I moved on to other things. He always cheered me on, always. I miss him and think of him dearly every day of my life. His words of love will ring on in my ear each day "I love you so much Bro."

My dad John, who has also passed on, has taught me to give everything I've got in whatever I do in life. Also, my sister Mary, my brother in law John and brother Johnny Jr. who have always said that I can do anything I wanted to and they would always be happy for me. Also, my three nieces, Regina, Jenna, and Elizabeth who always inspire me to be my best!

My many clients who have become great friends throughout this journey of love and commitment. Throughout the years along with many clients I have had to specialize workouts for each individuals needs. There were many. From a client suffering from Parkinsonism to one with Breast Cancer, and another from Open Heart Surgery. These clients and may I add friends have made me work my hardest to help them in becoming the best they can be through their hardships. May I add, there have been times that we have laughed about things in our lives and we have also cried many times in the midst of our tragedies. Too many and too hard to name.

But throughout these times, along with my family, my friends and new clients, we have strived to do our best. And I would like to dedicate many workouts in this book to the memories we have made together that will always keep a special place in my heart. I thank you and may GOD Bless each and everyone you and your families. Thank you for making my life so full.

I love you all so much!

Special thanks to Tina Colbert and Mary Rodriguez and all at Balboa Press who have helped me…

INTRODUCTION

As a young boy of two through the age of fifteen I was very scrawny and skinny. I also was anemic, and constantly sick. However, my dad, John, who was a competitive weightlifter, wouldn't hear of it. He wanted me to be strong and healthy. So, he bought me a set of water weights at the age of two and a half. Can you imagine me, practically a stick figure at the time, lifting weights? So, even through my years of poor health, I kept trying to be like my dad who was big and strong... and my hero.

By the age of 15, I went to work with my dad at his business, Johnny's Auto Body Shop. What a thrill it was to wake up every morning and know that, after school, I would be going to work alongside my hero. I remember the atmosphere was always pleasant there. My dad and his friends would tell their stories throughout the day, and at break time at 3pm we would stop and have coffee and snacks.

As the years went by, my brothers David and Johnny Jr. would come to work in the body shop with us. You could probably imagine that many times, there was more fun than work going on! But, that wasn't even the best part. On Tuesday and Thursday evenings, after dinner, we would drive back to the shop again. Only this time, it was to spend a few hours exercising in the back room where our dad built his very own gym. This is the place where I developed my inspiration and passion for coaching people to be their best selves. In the years to come, I studied very hard and became a Master Trainer with The National Federation of Professional Trainers (N.F.P.T.) along with this training and education I decided to become a Boxing Fitness Trainer as well as a Yoga Instructor.

Today, as a physical fitness trainer, my strong family values and precious memories influence my work. Since I was young, I was encouraged to believe in myself, and so I have always strived to help my clients do the same. I took on this particular project as a means to promote spiritual and physical health collectively.

This book is made up of 50 of my favorite workouts. The benefits of exercising are endless. I assure you, that whether you are just starting out or have stopped and decided to come back to training, you will feel so much better about yourself. It is a fact that exercise, even for 30 minutes a day will improve your physical strength, overall appearance, and help you feel better about yourself as the process will help your mind with chemical adjustments to your brain chemistry. It is a fact that many Psychiatrists and Therapists highly recommend exercise to help mood and depression in patients. I will tell you about that part of my life in another book at another time. Also, I have also included inspirational quotes at the top of each page of every workout, because I know that if your mind is right, then so will be your body. Plus, as a bonus, My wife Maria has put recipes for every part of your day, from breakfast to dinner.

Please think of this book of workouts, recipes, and quotes as a little piece of my heart from my Family. **For everyone who has ever tried and failed at every attempt at losing weight and obtaining a healthy lifestyle, this book is for you. As you train your body for the physical challenges necessary, please pay attention to the inspirational quotes. Sit quietly and meditate on them, and know that you are the hero of your own story.**

– Please go and make some beautiful memories with your family, friends, and loved ones!

God bless you!

WORKOUTS

WARNING:
Before starting any kind of exercise or physical routine, you are advised to consult your physician.

CAUTION:
There are workouts in this book that are meant for the athlete only (i.e. one who has been cross-training for more than 3 years).

All workouts apply to women as well as men. Use proper weight accordingly. For example, I warm up for about 7 minutes on the treadmill or recumbent bike, then go into my weight training workout. I squat with two 30 lb dumbbells for 10-12 reps then increase to 40 lb dumbbells for 8-10 reps.

BEGINNER WORKOUTS

> "You'll see it when you believe it"
>
> -Dr. Wayne Dyer

WORKOUT #1

Ultimate Chest and Back Workout with a Hint of Triceps and Biceps

Rest 2-3 minutes between each Superset

(A Superset is 2 or more exercises performed without a break. A Set is one exercise at a time with a minute break in between.)

Chest-back superset
Flat bench (chest and triceps, front shoulders) – 15 reps
Pulldown in front (back and biceps, rear shoulders) – 15 reps

Incline bench press (chest, tri's, front shoulders) – 12 reps
Pulldown or bent over row (back, bi's, rear shoulders) – 12 reps

Flat bench press (chest, tri's, shoulders) – 12 reps
Incline (upper chest, tri's, shoulders) – 12 reps

Pulldown (back and bi's) – 12 reps
Seated row (back and bi's, rear shoulders) – 12 reps

Flat bench (chest, tri's, shoulders) – 10 reps
15-25 Pushups (chest, tri's, shoulders, stomach)
10-15 Bent rows (back, bi's, shoulders)

Triceps pushdown – one set for 15 reps
Standing curls – one set for 15 reps

"A person is limited only by the thoughts that he chooses."

- James Allen, author of As a Man Thinketh

WORKOUT #2

Let's Plyometric!

(This is a bodyweight only workout.)

10 Burpees
10 Jumpers
25 Mountain climbers
10 Jumping squats
25 Crunches
25 Suitcases
10 Jumping squats
10 Burpees
10 Jumpers or frog jumps
10 Burpees

"A journey of a thousand miles begins with a single step."

- Confucius

WORKOUT #3

Back and Chest Workout with Plyometrics

Warm-up with 5-7 minutes on the treadmill, Stationary Bike etc. at low intensity and speed.

This workout will require you to rest between sets as needed.

- Pushups – 15-20 reps
- Bench press – 10 reps with light weight
- Pushups – 10 reps
- Bench press – 10 reps with medium weight
- Pushups – 15 reps
- Bench press – 10 reps with heavy weight
- Bench press – 25 reps with light to medium weight
- Pushups – 10-15 reps with feet on bench about 15.5 inches high

Then break for 2-3 minutes or when your heart rate is below 120bpm

- Bent over rows – 10 reps with light weight
- Pulldowns – 10 reps with medium weight
- Bent over rows – 10 reps with medium weight
- Pulldowns – 10 reps with medium weight
- Bent over rows – 10 reps with heavy weight
- Pulldowns – 10 reps with medium weight

Then rest 2-3 minutes.

Proceed to do:

- 25 Jumping jacks
- 10 Burpees
- 20 Mountain climbers
- 20 Jumpers

Take 25 grams of protein and perhaps a banana, as you need to replenish your glycogen stores!

> "Love who you are now because now is all you have."
>
> – Freddie Mangano

WORKOUT #4

Total Upper Body Workout

You may use dumbbells or barbells or mix it up as I do.

With this workout, use the same weight until you can increase in small amounts.

Chest-Shoulders-Triceps

1. Chest press – 15/12/15 reps
2. Pushups – 15 reps
3. Tricep pushdowns – 10/10/10 reps

Back-Biceps

1. Pulldowns – 15/12/10 reps
2. Bent rows – 15/12/10 reps
3. Curls – 10/10/10 reps

Shoulders

1. Press seated – 15/12/10 reps
2. Press standing – 10/20/30 reps
3. Upright rows – 10/12/15 reps

"Do the right thing and right things will happen."

– Freddie Mangano

WORKOUT #5

The "10-10-10"

1. 10 Sets of 10 pushups
2. 10 Light bench presses
3. 10 Sets of light bent rows

"Ask nothing, expect nothing, accept nothing. Today is the tomorrow I was so worried about yesterday."

- Anthony Hopkins

WORKOUT #6

Back-Chest Connection Training with Triceps and Biceps Superset

Warm up with dead-lift 2 sets.
Increase weight as needed and try to increase weight for every set.

1. Pulldowns superset with flat bench press; light weight for 12-15 reps.
2. Wide grip pulldowns; increase weight by 10 lbs.
3. Incline press; increase weight by 10-20 lbs.
4. Wide grip pull-downs 10 reps
5. Bent rows 10 reps
6. Flat bench press 10 reps
7. Incline press 10 reps
8. Low row 10 reps
9. Bent row 10 reps
10. Chest press 10 reps
11. Pushups 10 reps

Tri's and Bi's

1. Close grip benches with E-Z curl bar – 10 reps
2. Standing curl with E-Z curl bar – 10 reps
3. Triceps pushdowns – 12 reps
4. Standing dumbbell curls – 12 reps
5. Triceps pushdowns – 12 reps
6. E-Z curl bar – 12 reps

7. Triceps – 10 reps; take 10 lbs off / then 10 reps.
8. E-Z curl bar seated for 10 reps / then standing dumbbell curl for 10 reps.

Keep your focus each and every rep. Building muscle with every pump.

"Write your bad thoughts in the sand, and your good thoughts in cement."

- Unknown

WORKOUT #7

12 then 12 = 24... That's All

Warm up with a 7 minute walk.

Chest

1. 12 Flat benches
2. 12 Incline benches

Back

1. 12 Pulldowns
2. 12 Bent rows

Shoulders

1. Seated press – 12 reps
2. Standing press – 12 reps

Legs

1. Squats – 12 reps
2. Squats – 12 reps
3. Leg presses – 12 reps
4. Leg presses – 12 reps

Plyometrics, if you can!

1. 12 Navy seals
2. 12 Jumpers
3. 12 Navy seals
4. 12 Mountain climbers

WORKOUT #8

Leg Intensity Workout with Upper Body

Warm up as usual with about 7 minutes of aerobic; not too intense!

1. Squat-clean-press – 15 lbs for 15 reps.
    Superset with seated press for 15 reps with medium weight.

Then:

2. Seated leg press – 50 to 100 lbs for 15 reps.
    Superset with pulldowns for 15 reps.
    Superset with curls for 15 reps.

3. Leg curls / squats / leg presses for 15 reps and as heavy as you can take it.
4. Chest press for 3 sets of 15 reps progressing weight.

"Treat yourself with respect; Others will do the same!

– Freddie Mangano

WORKOUT #9

Chest-Shoulders-Triceps

Warm up with 5-7 minutes of aerobics.

1. Shoulder press 10 lbs for 10 reps.
2. Shoulder press 10 lbs for 10 reps.
3. Shoulder press 10 lbs for 12 reps.

Rest for 1-2 minutes

4. Tricep pushdowns for 10 lbs for 10 reps.
5. Tricep pushdowns for 10 lbs for 10 reps.
6. Tricep pushdowns for 10 lbs for 12 reps.

Rest for 1-2 minutes

7. Pushups for 10 reps.
8. Chest press for 10 reps.
9. Incline chest press for 10 reps.
10. Chest press for 10 reps.

INTERMEDIATE WORKOUTS

WORKOUT #10

Kettlebell Workout

Warm up with 15 reps of swings.

1. Squat roll for 10 reps (holding kettlebell in crank position, squat down, sit on the mat and roll back on your spine. Then, come forward to come up again into the standing position. Repeat for 9 more reps).
2. Squat press for 10 reps.
3. Kettlebell Swings for 10 reps each side.
4. Windmill for 10 reps each side.
5. 2-Hand swing with medium weight kettlebell in each hand.
6. Kettlebell swing with heavy weight for 15 reps.
7. Squat–clean–press with kettlebell for 15 reps.

Repeat this 3x around (If you are exhausted after one time around, Stop!)

WORKOUT #11

Upper Body Workout

Warmup 5-7 Minutes with light intensity aerobics

Back:

1. Deadlift with Olympic bar and medium weight for 10 reps; 2 sets for a warm–up.
2. Deadlift with heavier weight for 10 reps.
3. Low row with medium weight for 10 reps.
4. Pullovers with medium weight for 10 reps.

Chest:

1. Flat bench press with medium weight for 12 reps.
2. Incline bench press with heavier weight for 12 reps.
3. Pushups for 25 reps.

Shoulders:

1. Seated press for 12 reps with medium weight.
2. Standing side raises for 12 reps with light weight (one foot forward slightly bent and don't raise the weight above parallel).
3. Upright rows for 12 reps with medium weight (if you have a shoulder injury, as do some of my clients, please defer to the shrug with heavier weight if you can handle it – but be careful and mindful if you have an injury. Safety always comes first!).

Triceps:

1. Pushdowns for 12 reps with medium weight.
2. Lying triceps extensions for 12 reps.
3. Close grip pushups for 12 reps.

Biceps:

1. Seated dumbbell curls for 12 reps with medium weight.
2. Standing E-Z curl bar curls for 12 reps with heavy weight.
3. Standing dumbbell curls for 12 reps with heavy weight.

Between each body part, make it interesting and throw in some plyometrics for 10 to 20 reps (I would do 10 burpees, 20 mountain climbers and 20 jumpers between each body part).

"The purpose of our lives is to be happy."

- Dalai Lama

WORKOUT #12

The 12-24-36

(This is an upper body workout only.)

The intensity of this workout is all-encompassing!

Focus on doing the moves very strictly and place your mind on this (and only this) workout!

Warm up with 12 reps of the weight you will start with in the Bench Press.

Use a weight you can do the total amount of reps with. Slower and lighter is better!

So here goes:

Chest-Triceps-Shoulders

1. Bench press – 12 reps
2. Tricep pushdowns – 24 reps
3. Incline bench press – 36 reps
   Now wait for up to 1 minute, then we will proceed to make up another 36 reps with 12 reps each of the same exercises above (see below).

1. Bench press – 12 reps
2. Tricep pushdowns – 12 reps
3. Incline bench press – 12 reps

Back-Biceps-Shoulders

1. Bent rows with dumbbells or barbell – 12 reps
2. Standing curls – 24 reps
3. Pulldowns – 36 reps
   Rest 1 minute.

1. Bent rows – 12 reps
2. Standing curls – 12 reps
3. Pulldowns – 12 reps

Shoulders

1. Seated shoulder press – 12 reps
2. Standing side raises – 24 reps
3. Upright rows – 36 reps

Rest for 30 seconds.

1. Seated shoulder press – 12 reps
2. Standing side raises – 12 reps
3. Upright rows – 12 reps

> "Your big opportunity may be right where you are now."
>
> - Napoleon Hill

WORKOUT #13

HIIT Training

Everything for weight training is 2 supersets and medium weight.

Weight Training:

Bench press – 10 reps / pulldowns – 10 reps

Plyometrics:

25 Jumping jacks / 15 navy seals / 25 push-ups / 15 bent rows / 25 punches / 15 kicks / 50 punches

Weight Training:

Leg presses – 10 reps / shoulders presses – 10 reps / squats – 10 reps / upright rows – 10 reps

Plyometrics:

50 Runners / 20 jumpers / 10 navy seals

Weights Training:

Tricep pulldowns – 10 reps / biceps curls – 10 reps

Plyometrics:

25 Kicks on heavy bag / 50 punches

"Don't watch the clock; do what it does. Keep going."

- Sam Levenson

WORKOUT #14

The "20's"

20 Squats / 20 bent rows / 20 leg presses / 20 shoulder presses / 20 leg presses

Plyos:

50 Punches / 10 kicks / 50 punches / 40 jumping jacks

Weights:

Chest presses – 10 reps of 20 lb, 30 lb, 40 lb, and 50 lb dumbbells; then 10-20 pushups.

Bent rows – 10 reps with 30's and 40's.

Squat rows – 10-20 reps (this needs to be done on a cable machine) or just squat.

Plyos:

20 Side kicks / 10 front kicks / 50 punches / 20 side kicks / 40 jumping jacks / 50 runners / 20 navy seals

Weights:

20 Shoulder presses / 20 curls / 20 tri's / 20 squats / 25 boxer crunches
2 Rounds of boxing for 2-3 minutes each
Squats – 10 reps / leg presses – 10 reps / leg curls – 10 reps

Plyos:

20 Jumping jacks / 25-50 punches / 10 kicks / 25 suitcases

"Fall seven times, stand up eight."

- Japanese Proverb

WORKOUT #15

Plyos and Weights Forever

50 Pushups / 50 jumping jacks / 20 navy seals / 20 jumpers / 50 runners

Weights:

Chest press superset with leg press – 2 sets of 20 reps each

Plyos:

25 Jumping jacks / 10 navy seals / 50 runners

Weights:

Bent rows superset with shoulder press

Plyos:

100 punches, then 25 front kicks each.

Weights:

(2x around as a circuit)
20 Reps of tri's
20 Squats
20 Reps of bi's

Plyos:

40 Jumping jacks / 10 navy seals / 20 jumpers / 25 kicks / 50 punches

"There is only one happiness in this life, to love and be loved."

- George Sand

WORKOUT #16

The Plyo Weight Training Workout

Warm up with 50 jumping jacks and 25 navy seals.

- Squat-clean-press: 15 reps 2x, with 30-second rest in between.

Then wait 2 minutes.

- Leg presses for 15 reps, superset / pull-downs for 15 reps, superset / curls for 15 reps 3x.

Then wait 1-2 minutes.

- Curls superset with shoulder presses 2x for 15 reps.

Then wait 1 minute.

- Leg presses for 15 reps, superset / squats for 15 reps 3x around.

Then:

- Chest presses for 12 reps, superset / flyes for 10 reps 3x around.
- Finish off with 25 suitcases.

"Those who leave everything in God's Hand will eventually see God's Hand in everything."

- Unknown

WORKOUT #17

Calisthenics-Plyometrics

1. Planks for 30 seconds / front-side-side.
2. Bulgarian sandbag – 2 sets / snatch and squat – 10 reps.
3. 30-second drills of jumping jacks / Bulgarian sandbag squats – 2-3 sets.

Take a 2-3 minute break.

4. Jumping jacks – 25 reps / squats with 10-15 lb sandbag
5. Mountain climbers – 50 reps

> "Unhappy people are contagious, stay away from them."
>
> - Chazz Palminteri

WORKOUT #18

Total Body Workout with Plyometrics

Warmup on treadmill or bike (or any aerobic will do as long as it is not too intense and only lasts for 5-7 minutes) to warm up the lungs and heart to get the body ready for the workout.

1. Chest, shoulders, triceps: 10-10-20 reps / chest press and incline chest press (alternate exercises).
2. Back, biceps, shoulders: 10-10-20 reps / bent over rows, pulldowns, low rows – 10-10-20 reps
3. Shoulders and triceps with plyometrics: 10-10-20 reps / shoulder presses and side raises (alternate back and forth with each) / 25-50 jumping jacks and 25 navy seal pushups.
4. Legs: 10-10-20 reps / squats, leg presses, leg curls (have fun with these, as you may go from switching the first exercise to the last and so on).
5. Back, again: 10-10-20 reps / bent rows only heavy to light weight.
6. Biceps: 10-10-20 reps / curls with E-Z curl bar and dumbbells (choose your weight carefully; you are already warmed up and somewhat fatigued from the previous exercises).

Now finish off with plyometrics of 50 jumping jacks, 10 front kicks each leg into a heavy bag, and 50 more jumping jacks.

Then, get 20 to 30 grams of protein from a shake with perhaps ½ of a banana.

"God will provide the ladder of your pit of problems, but you must be willing to climb up."

- Christian Associates

WORKOUT #19

HIIT Training

Warm up with 25 jumping jacks and 10 burpees for 3x around.

- Rotation with barbell (which means you place on one end of a barbell a 10-25 or higher plate, then you position the other end - which has no plate on it - in a corner with a towel, or just push it tight against the corner so it is secure) – 10 reps.

With the bar in front of you, grab bar at plate end and lift it up to your chest, then lift it above your head and rotate it halfway from one shoulder to the other, going from left to right in an arc or sort of a half moon.

- 10 Second plate hold (hold a 10-25-45 lb plate straight out with your locked out arms for 10 seconds).
- Circle plate (hold the same plate and create circles from forehead to belly button 10x around one way, then 10x the other way) – 10 reps around each way.
- Dumbbell squats with one arm press – 10 reps each side.
- Jumping squats – 10 reps {Bodyweight}
- Jumping jacks – 20 reps
- Navy seals Pushups – 10 reps
- Side kicks in a heavy bag or in the air – 10 reps.
- 30 Second to 1 minute of punches in a heavy bag (if you don't have a heavy bag, no worries, just punch into the air).

"Life is short. Do more of what makes you happy."

- Life Quotes

WORKOUT #20

Full Body Plyometrics

Okay, now this is an interval workout, which means you do 30 seconds of each exercise, then rest for 1 minute 30 seconds, then back to another 30 seconds of work.

1. Squat jumps – 30 seconds
2. Mountain climbers – 30 seconds
3. Squats with twists – 30 seconds
4. Crunches – 30 seconds
5. Alternating arms and leg raises – 30 seconds

1 minute rest.

Then:

6. Squat – 30 seconds
7. Jumping jacks – 30 seconds

1 minute 30 second rest, then repeat 1 through 5.

1 minute 30 second rest, then repeat 6 and 7.

"Trust yourself, you know more than you think."

- Benjamin Spock

WORKOUT #21

Aerobic and Plyometric

Warm up for 5-7 minutes.

- Squat jumps – 10 reps
- Rope jumps – 30 seconds
- Burpees – 30 seconds
- Step-ups – 17 to 25 inches high onto bench or box for 30 seconds each side.

Repeat for 3-5 times around.

"You can't undo the actions others did to you, but you can choose to let it go and let God heal it."

- Darling of God

WORKOUT #22

Lower Body with Aerobic Intensity

Warm up for 7 minutes.

1. Squat jumps – 10 reps
   Superset with: jumping jacks – 25 reps.

2. Jump rope for 1 minute.
   Superset with: burpees – 15 reps.

3. Step-ups onto 20-inch bench or box for 10 reps each leg.
   Superset with: jumps onto box or bench for 10 jumps.
   Superset with: jumping jacks – 25 reps.

4. 100 punches into heavy bag with mitts or training gloves.
   Superset with: shoulder press – 25 reps.

5. 100 punches again as above.
   Superset with: bent rows – 25 reps with light weight.

"That which does not kill us makes us stronger"

–Friedrich Nietzsche

WORKOUT #23

Upper Body and Plyometrics

Warm up with about a 7 minute low intensity aerobic move.

This is another type of plyometric workout, but it's also a weight training workout:

1. Flat bench press for 15 reps with light to medium weight.
2. Pushups for 25 to 30 reps.
   Then, 50 jumping jacks.
   Repeat this circuit 2x, adding weight each time.

3. Pulldowns for 15 reps with medium to heavy weight.
4. Bent rows for 15 reps with heavy weight (you may use dumbbells, barbells, or kettlebells).
   Then, 25 jumping squats.
   Repeat this 2x as well.

5. Squats for 15 reps with medium to heavy weight.
6. Leg press for 15 reps with medium weight.
   Then, 50 runners and 25 jumpers.
   This is repeated 2x.

WORKOUT #24

Leg Day Workout

(This is a bodyweight only workout.)

Start with an aerobic warm-up.

1. Squat for 10 reps.
2. Squat for 20 reps.
3. Squat for 30 reps.
4. Leg press for 30 reps.
5. Leg press for 20 reps.
6. Leg press for 10 reps.
7. Jumping jacks for 50 reps.
8. Squat jumps for 10 reps.
9. Runners for 50 reps.
10. Jumpers for 30 reps.
11. Squats for 10 reps.
12. Leg press for 10 reps.

> "There is little success where there is little laughter"
>
> –Andrew Carnegie

WORKOUT #25

Chest and Back Workout

To all women or men who cannot lift the weight in any of these workouts, please adjust your weight accordingly. Remember, it's not how heavy you lift, it's the form.

Low-impact aerobic warm-up for 5 minutes.

1. Bench press for 15 reps with light weight.
2. Incline press for 15 reps.
3. 25-30 Pushups
4. 50 Jumping jacks

Rest 30 seconds.

5. Bench press for 15 reps with medium or heavy weight.
6. Pullovers for 15 reps.
7. 50 runners

Rest 20 seconds.

8. Bench press for 10 reps.
9. 25 Pushups and 50 jumpers

Rest 1 minute.

Incline press for 10 reps.

10. Pulldowns for 12 reps.
11. Bent rows for 12 reps.

Rest 10 seconds.

12. Bent rows for 12 reps.
13. Pulldowns for 12 reps.
14. Bent rows for 12 reps.
15. Pulldowns for 12 reps.

Rest 1 minute.

16. Seated incline curls – 25 to 30 lbs each hand (alternate for one rep each then together for one rep to 10 reps total).
17. Standing curls with 40 lb dumbbells for one rep; then go down to 30 lb dumbbells in each hand for one rep; repeat as follows for 10 reps total.

This is the end of the workout. Please remember to take in a 25-30 gram protein drink afterward.

"I can accept failure, but I cannot accept not trying."

- Michael Jordan

WORKOUT #26

Legs Only

Warning: This workout is not for those who cannot do plyometrics!

Warm up with 2 sets of 10 jumping squats.

1. Squats for 20 reps.
2. Leg press for 20 reps.
3. Squats for 20 reps.
4. Leg press for 20 reps (10 reps each leg).
5. Squats for 20 reps.
6. Leg press for 20 reps.
7. Leg curls for 20 reps.
8. Calf raises for 20 reps (4x).
9. 10 Kicks into a heavy bag (2x).

"A Goal is a dream with a deadline"

–Napoleon Hill

WORKOUT #27

Total Body with Core Training

Warm up with 5-7 minutes of low-impact aerobics.

These can be performed on an incline of about 12 inches:

- 15 Reverse crunches
- 15 Leg raises
- 15 Reverse crunches

These may be done on an incline of about 25-30 inches:

- 10 Reverse crunches
- 10 Leg raises
- 10 Reverse crunches

- 12 Incline bench presses
- 24 Flat benches
- 12 Incline benches

Rest.

- 12 Pulldowns
- 24 Low rows
- 12 Bent rows

Rest.

- 24 Shoulder presses
- 24 Tricep pushdowns
- 24 Curls

Rest.

If you are feeling strong, continue with legs:

- 12 Leg presses
- 24 Squats
- 36 Leg presses performed in this fashion – 12 leg presses / 12 single leg presses / 12 leg presses.

ADVANCED

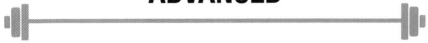

"The hardest work you'll do in this life is the work you do on yourself."

- Freddie Mangano

WORKOUT #28

Killer Legs

1. Squats for 10 reps with light weight – i.e. 10-20 lb dumbbells.
2. Squats for 10 reps – 30 lb dumbbells.
3. Squats for 10 reps – 35 lb dumbbells.
4. Squats for 10 reps – 40 lb dumbbells.
5. Leg press for 12 reps.
6. Calf raises for 25 reps.

Rest 1 minute.

7. Leg press for 12 reps.
8. Leg press for 10 reps.
9. Squats for 10 reps – heavy weight.
10. Squats for 10 reps – 10 lbs lighter weight.
11. Squats for 10 reps – 10 lbs lighter weight.
12. Repeat the second circuit one more time, and then go home!

"Do the thing you fear, and fear will disappear."

- Ralph Waldo Emerson

WORKOUT #29

Ultimate Leg and Plyometric Day with a Washboard Abs Workout

1. 10 Leg presses with jumping squats
2. 10 Leg curls (if you are not near a leg machine, replace these with squats).

Repeat 1 and 2 – 2-3x.

Then:

Squats – 10 reps with dumbbells.

Then:

Repeat 1 and 2 again.

Plyometrics:

30 Jumpers
50 Mountain climbers (runners)

Stomach:

Incline weight crunches: 2 sets with weight approx. 10-15 lbs for women and 20-25 lbs for men (hold a dumbbell on your chest with 2 hands, have your feet secured, and crunch up).

> "Success is not final. Failure is not fatal. It is the courage to go on that counts."
>
> - Sir Winston Churchill

WORKOUT #30

The 40's

Warm up with a light weight, with a squat, chest press, and bent row for 12 reps each.

Then:

> Flat bench press – 40 reps with moderate weight.
> Bent row – 40 reps with moderate weight.
> Squats – 20 reps with moderate weight.
> Leg press – 20 reps
> Calf raises – 40 reps
> Tricep pushdown – 40 reps
> Standing curls – 40 reps
> Shoulder press – 40 reps
> Pushups – 40 reps
> V-ups – 40 reps

Okay, now on a day like this, please don't do anything else like aerobics, plyometrics, etc.

You are done!

Now you can go have some fun!

> "Once you make a decision, the universe conspires to make it happen."
>
> - Ralph Waldo Emerson

WORKOUT #31

Upper Body Ultimate (Extremely Advanced!)

Now if the 40's was a workout you think you could do, take a look at this one!

Chest:

Bench press – 25 reps - 30 reps - 40 reps

Back:

Bent row – 25 reps, then low row 30 reps, then pulldowns 40 reps.

Shoulders:

Seated press – 25 reps - 30 reps - 40 reps

Triceps:

Extensions – 40 reps

Biceps:

Curls – 40 reps
(That's 380 reps!)
Crunches – 3 sets of 10 reps on an incline.
Reverse crunches – 3 sets of 10 reps on an incline.

"They can conquer who believe they can."

- Ralph Waldo Emerson

WORKOUT #32

Leg Workout with Plyometrics

Warm up with Roman deadlifts for 2 sets of 10 reps.

Here's the workout:

1. Squat-clean-press (6x).
2. Jump squats for 10 reps.
3. Squat-clean-press (5x).
4. Burpees for 10 reps.
5. Squats for 10 reps.
6. Mountain climbers for 25 reps.
7. Squats for 10 reps.
8. Jumping jacks for 25 reps, burpees for 10 reps, then mountain climbers for 10 reps.

Drink plenty of water and a protein drink of 25-30 grams.

> "We make a living by what we get, but we make a life by what we give."
>
> - Winston Churchill

WORKOUT #33

Full Body with Plyos

- Squats – 10 reps with 10 lbs
- Squats – 10 reps with 15 lbs
- 10 Jumping squats
- 25 Jumping jacks
- Squats – 10 reps with 15 lbs
- Squats – 10 reps with 10 lbs
- 15 Jumping squats
- 50 Jumping jacks
- 40 Leg presses
- Upper body bent row – 10 reps with 15 lbs
- Incline press – 20 reps with 15 lbs
- Shoulder press – 30 reps with 12-15 lbs
- 20 Burpees
- Triceps pushdowns – 40 reps
- 25 Jumping jacks
- Standing bicep curls – 40 reps
- 25 Jumping jacks
- 25 Leg raises
- 25 Boxer crunches

Drink an extra quart of water on the days of training with weights, as well as your aerobic day.

"Sometimes things become possible if we want them bad enough." -

T.S. Eliot

WORKOUT #34

Plyometrics Circuit Training

Circuit #1 – non-stop if you can handle it!

1. 25 Jumping jacks
2. 10 Burpees
3. 10 High jumps onto a 15.5 foot box or bench.

This repeats 3x around. Rest time is 1-3 minutes between circuits. RHR of 120 bpm or lower before returning to the next circuit.

Circuit #2

1. 20 Jumpers
2. 20 Double jumps from ground to a stepper to a box or bench
3. 10 Kettlebell swings
4. 10 Squats with kettlebell (15 to 20 lbs).

This repeats 2x around (you may wait 1-2 minutes between this circuit).

Always remember that your heart rate should be at 120 bpm or below as your recovery heart rate!

Circuit #3

1. 20 Double jumps forward and back.
2. 10 Side-to-side kettlebell swings
3. 10 Jumpers
4. 25 Mountain climbers

This goes 2x around if you can handle it. If not, you can do it just once. I promise, no one will call you a baby after this circuit!

Take in a protein drink and plenty of water.

This takes approximately 23-25 minutes and burns about 400-450 calories.

"A river cuts through rock, not because of its power, but because of its persistence."

- Jim Watkins

WORKOUT #35

Kettlebells

1. Kettlebell swings – 10 swings for a warm-up.
2. 10 Swings with a light weight.
3. 10 Swings side-to-side with a medium weight.
4. 15 Squats with a heavy weight, holding the kettlebell in the crank position (by the sides of the handle).
5. 25 Jumping jacks
6. 15 Jump squats with a 10 lb kettlebell.

Rest for 1-2 minutes.

Now we are going up and down the rack:

1. Low weight kettlebell swings – 15 reps.
2. Medium weight swings – 15 reps.
3. Heavy weight swings – 15 reps.
4. Squats for 15 reps, holding the heavy weight kettlebell.
5. Kettlebell swings side-to-side for 10 reps each side.
6. 50 Jumping jacks

Rest for 1-2 minutes.

Repeat the second circuit one more time.

WORKOUT #36

Lower Body

Warm up with leg presses for 2 sets of 10 reps.

Then, 1 set of Romanian deadlifts for 12 reps.

1. Squats – 4 sets of progressive squats (meaning increasing the weight for approx. 10-20 lbs each set).
2. Leg presses – 5 sets of: 10-12-15-20-25 reps, adding 10-25 lbs each set.
3. Step ups with a dumbbell in each hand on a 15 to 17 inch bench- 4 sets of 5-10-12-15 reps, adding weight for each set
4. Leg curls – 4 sets of 15 reps, adding weight as heavy as you can stand it, without compromising form.
5. Squats – 3 sets of 12 reps with medium weight.

It's Leg Day, so stop crying and do the workout! (Then cry afterward... as I always do!)

"The only way to have a friend is to be one."

- Ralph Waldo Emerson

WORKOUT #37

Lower Body Plyos Mixed with Full Body

Walk on treadmill for about 5-7 minutes to warm-up.

Then:

1. 10 Jump squats
2. Kettlebell side-to-side swings
3. Jumping jacks for 50 reps.
4. 10 Squat jumps
5. Jump rope for 1 minute.
6. Burpees for 10 reps.
7. 10 Step-ups on a 15-17 inch box or bench with 10 lbs in each hand.

Repeat circuit 2-3 times.

WORKOUT #38

Legs: 12-24-36 (Now, this is grueling!)

Warm up with back extensions.

1. Squats – 12 reps
2. Leg curls – 24 reps
3. Squats – 36 reps

Rest 1-2 minutes.

1. Leg press – 36 reps
2. Squats – 12 reps
3. Leg curls – 24 reps

Follow up with 2 sets of 12 jumping squats (if your body and mind will allow).

You may repeat this circuit 2x if you feel strong and if you are not training the next day, but I wouldn't advise doing more than 2x around if done correctly.

"When I stand before God at the end of my life, I would hope that I would not have a single bit of talent left and could say, I used everything you gave me."

- Erma Bombeck

WORKOUT #39

Circuit Training

Every circuit is 3x around.

Circuit #1

1. Weight navy seals (burpees) – 10 reps, 3x around.

Circuit #2

1. Flat bench press – 10 reps.
2. Pushups – 10 reps, and then runners – 20 reps (be sure to do between 1. And 3.).
3. Incline press – 10 reps

Circuit #3

1. Heavy bent rows – 10 reps
2. Navy seals (burpees) – 10 reps
3. Triceps – 10 reps
4. Jumpers – 20 reps
5. Standing curls – 15 reps
6. Jumping jacks – 50 reps

> "Do not fear going forward slowly; fear only to stand still."
>
> - Chinese Proverb

WORKOUT #40

"The Blaster"

Each circuit is 3 supersets.

Chest-Triceps-Shoulders

1.   Pushups – 25 reps superset with:
     a) Bench press – 25 reps.

Rest 1-2 minutes between sets and circuits.

Be sure to do 2nd superset with heavier weight.

Back-Biceps-Shoulders

1.   Low Row – 10 reps superset with:
     a) High row – 10 reps.
     b) Bent row – 10 reps.

"The way to get started is to quit talking and begin doing."

- Walt Disney

WORKOUT #41

Quick and Fierce Workouts

The "10 for 10"

1. 10 Squats bodyweight only!
2. 10 Navy seals (burpees)

Do this circuit for 5-10x around.

"Without Inspiration the best powers of the mind remain dormant. There is a fuel in us which needs to be ignited with sparks."

– Johann Gottfried Von Herder

WORKOUT #42

The "50"

1. 50 Medicine ball throws, either feet-against-feet with a partner or up against the wall.

Then:

1. 50 Squats with light weight dumbbells.
2. 50 Leg presses with light to medium weight.

Note: You may also break this up with 25 reps/Rest/25 reps

"One Good Thing about music, when it hits you, you feel no pain."

– Bob Marley

WORKOUT #43

Your Optimal Health LLC Advanced Workout

Warning: You must work up to this one slowly and steadily

Circuit #1

1. Tricep extensions – 50 reps
2. Squats – 50 reps
3. 75 Bench presses, flat or inclined
4. 10 Navy seals, with 10x running up and down 14 steps.

Circuit #2

1. Low rows – 50 reps.
2. Curls – 50 reps
3. Leg presses – 75 reps
4. Stairs 10x
5. 60 Crunches / 60 reverse crunches

> "Only those who dare to fail greatly can ever achieve greatly."
>
> - Robert Kennedy

WORKOUT #44

Legs-Back-Chest

This workout will be 15 reps for the first circuit, 12 reps for the second circuit, and 10 reps for the third circuit. Try it without resting, but no worries if you need to take a break!

The 3rd round is optional.

1. Squats
2. Leg presses
3. Bent row
4. Chest press
5. Shoulder press
6. Upright rows
7. Lying down triceps
8. Seated curls
9. Leg curls

"Train up a child in the way he should go; and when he is old, he will not depart from it."

- Proverbs 22:6

WORKOUT 45

Let's Box

Warm-up with 50 Jumping jacks.

    15 Navy seals
    25 Jumpers
    50 Mountain climbers
    50 Punches on a heavy bag.
    10 Front kicks, each leg.

Repeat 2x.

Then:

Standing Speed Bag Punches

    100 Left and rights

Then:

    25 Lefts
    25 Rights
    50 Lefts and rights

Heavy Bag Punches

> 100 Speed punches
> 100 Hard punches
> 100 Speed punches
> 100 Hard punches
> 60 Boxer crunches

Jump rope for 3 minutes.

Now go home!

"Choose a job you love, and you will never have to work a day in your life."

- Confucius

WORKOUT #46

Kettlebells

Warm-up with a brisk walk for about 7 minutes.

1. Figure 8's for 5 reps each way. With a kettlebell as heavy as you can endure you will be doing figure 8's (holding in the crank position, which means holding the kettlebell by the sides of the handle).
2. Squats for 10 reps with heavy kettlebell.
3. Get-ups on knees – 10 reps each side.
4. 2-Hand up and back for abdominals (with knees bent and lying on your back, start with kettlebell held in crank position behind your head on floor or bench, then come into a crunch position and push the kettlebell through the opening in your bent knees) – 10 reps.

Do these as circuits; 2 to 3 circuits around.

WORKOUT #47

Plyometrics with Core Training and Calisthenics

Warm up with 5 minutes of low-impact aerobics.

1. Farmer's walk (holding weights above your head) with 10 to 25 lbs in each hand, and walk 40 yards).
2. Suitcase walk (with weight by your sides) for 2 minutes.
3. Racked position walk (with weights close to your shoulders) for 1 minute.
4. 50 Jumping jacks
5. 50 Jumpers
6. 20 Squats
7. 20 Pushups
8. 20 Bench presses
9. 20 Pulldowns
10. 20 Reverse crunches
11. 20 Triceps pushdowns
12. 20 Leg raises
13. 20 Standing curls
14. 50 Runners
15. 20 Shoulder presses

Take in 20 to 30 grams of protein after your workout.

"Act as if what you do makes a difference. It does."

- William James

WORKOUT #48

Plyometrics with Core Training

Warm up with 7 minutes of low-impact aerobics only.

1. 25 Mountain climbers
2. 25 Frog jumps
3. 25 Navy seal pushups
4. Pushups (as many as you can do) up to 50.
   Repeat 1x, then rest 1-2 minutes.

5. Squats bodyweight only for 25 reps.
6. Boxer crunches for 25 reps.
7. Suitcases for 25 reps.
8. Squats for 25 reps.
   Repeat 1x then rest 1-2 minutes.
   Then do 1 through 6 as a circuit.

WORKOUT #49

Legs with Back and Shoulders and Plyometrics

Warm up for 5-7 minutes with low-impact aerobics.

1. Leg raises for 10 reps with both legs; then 10 reps on each leg.
2. Shoulder press for 10 reps, and then each arm for 10 reps.
3. Pulldowns for 15 reps – underhand grip shoulder width.
4. Leg raises (same as Step 1).
5. Bent rows – three sets nonstop for 10 reps for 3 different weights (20's, 30's, 40's).
6. Squats – three sets nonstop with 25, 30, 40 lb dumbbells.

Plyometrics: runners, jumpers, burpees – 25 each.

Repeat circuit 1-2 times around.

"The world is a book, and those who do not travel read only a page."

- Saint Augustine

WORKOUT #50

Full Body Workout: The 10-12-20 Plyometric

Warm up with 7 minutes of low-impact aerobics.

Chest press for 10-12-20 reps 2x.

Add them together and do 42 reps of jumping jacks.

Bent row for 10-12-20 reps 2x.

Again, do 42 reps of runners.

Shoulder press for 10-12-20 reps 2x.

Do 42 reps of pushups.

Squats for 10-12-20 reps.

Do 42 reps of frog kicks.

Leg press for 10-12-20 reps.

Do 42 reps of jumping jacks.

Standing bicep curls for 10-12-20 reps.

Do 42 reps of runners.

Tricep pushdowns for 10-12-20 reps.

Do 42 reps of reverse crunches.

"I would rather walk with GOD in the dark than go alone in the light."

- Mary Gardiner Brainard

RECOMMENDED PRE- AND POST-WORKOUT MEALS

PRE-WORKOUT MEAL

(Approximately 1-2 hours before heavy weight training)

1. Peanut butter and jelly on 1 or 2 slices of whole wheat bread, with a glass of whole milk, almond milk, or water.

POST-WORKOUT MEAL

(Within 45 minutes after workout to restore glycogen into muscle tissue)

Mix 8 oz. of water or almond milk with 20-30 grams of your favorite whey protein powder.

RECIPES

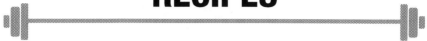

BREAKFAST

Recipe 1:
Oatmeal and Egg White Delight

½ cup of oatmeal with half of a banana, topped with cinnamon. On the side, cook 3-4 egg whites (you can add a little ketchup if you'd like). Be sure to drink 16 oz. of water after your meal.

Recipe 2:
Egg White Sandwich

1. Spray Pam in a pan.
2. 2 egg whites and 1 egg, scrambled.
3. Put on flatbread or bread of your choice (can be toasted).
4. Add ketchup, if desired for taste.

Protein - 14 grams
Carbohydrates - 20 grams
Fats - 5 grams

Recipe 3:
Protein Oatmeal Pancakes

1/2 cup dry oats (quick oats are best) cooked with water
Add 1 egg and 1 egg white.
Add 1 scoop of whey protein (any flavor).
Add sweetener to taste (honey, Stevia, or Splenda).
Add cinnamon to taste.
Add berries if desired.
Mix cooked oats with the remaining ingredients until you have the consistency of pancake batter (you may have to add water or oats to achieve the correct consistency).

Scoop pancake batter into hot skillet sprayed with Pam.

Makes 4-6 pancakes.

Recipe 4:
Fresh Vegetable Scramble

⅔ cup of dried vegetables (use a variety, i.e. zucchini, peppers, broccoli, onions, asparagus, spinach, etc.)

1 whole egg and 2 egg whites whisked together

Salt and pepper to taste

Spray Pam in a pan.
Sauté veggies in pan until softened to taste.
Add salt and pepper.
Add in whisked eggs.
Scramble together.
Serve with wheat toast or English muffin.

Recipe 5:
Protein-packed Cheerios

1 cup Cheerios
6-8 oz. almond milk
20 grams protein powder
Combine Cheerios with protein powder, then add almond milk to the cereal.

LUNCH

Recipe 1:
Tuna Sandwich

Open up a can or two of chunk white tuna, put into a bowl, and mix it with one teaspoon of mayo and one teaspoon of dark mustard (also one teaspoon of relish if you want a little sweetness). Put it between 2 slices of whole wheat bread and have a great meal with 26 to 30 grams of protein and 25 grams of carbohydrates. Also, the good fats from the tuna will be appreciated by your heart, your joints (for lubrication), and your brain!

Recipe 2:
Avocado Tuna Salad

1 can of solid white tuna (in water)
1/2 avocado
1 teaspoon of light mayonnaise (optional)
Diced onion and/or celery to taste (optional)
Salt and pepper to taste
2 cups mixed salad

Drain tuna.
Add avocado and light mayonnaise to tuna and mix well.
Add onion, celery, salt and pepper to taste.
Toss mixed salad with tuna mixture.

Recipe 3:
Grilled Chicken and Kale Salad

2 chicken breasts grilled to perfection
1 bowl of kale salad

1/2 cup balsamic vinaigrette
1 tablespoon olive oil
4 strawberries cut into halves

Cut chicken breasts into bite-size pieces.
Blend strawberries with balsamic vinegar and oil.
Mix into salad.

Makes 2-3 servings.

Recipe 4
Easy Protein Bowl

2 Hard Eggs Sliced
½ Cup Cooked Turkey or Chicken Cubed
½ Cup Black Beans
½ Cup Chick Peas (Garbanzo Beans)
½ Cup Cooked Broccoli

Begin with Broccoli and Layer bottom of the bowl
Layer all other ingredients, ending with sliced hard boiled eggs
Add 2-3 Tablespoons of your favorited low fat dressing

Recipe 5
Honey Balsamic Chicken and Vegetables

Ingredients:

1 Large Boneless Chicken Breast (pound it out evenly and cut into cubes)
1 Steamable Bag of Broccoli Florets
½ medium onion sliced
1 Red Pepper sliced
3 -4 Tablespoons of Balsamic Vinegar and ½ teaspoon of honey combined
3 Tablespoons of Vegetable based oil

Non-Stick Cooking Spray
Salt and Pepper

In a pan, saute onions and peppers with one tablespoon of oil and cooking spray until tender.
Salt and Pepper to taste.
Heat broccoli bag according to instruction
Salt and Pepper to taste

Transfer all cooked vegetables to a bowl and set aside.

In the same vegetable pan, add 2 tablespoons of oil and saute chicken until cooked through.
Salt and Pepper to taste.

Add vegetables to cooked chicken along with Balsamic Vinegar and Honey.

Mix thoroughly and heat an additional 1-2 minutes (add more or less balsamic vinegar/honey to taste)

Serve alone or with Brown Rice or with side salad

DINNER

Recipe 1:
Grilled Chicken Breasts with Spinach and a Baked Sweet Potato

1. Grill 2 chicken breasts in a pan. First pound breasts to tenderize, season with salt, pepper and Mrs. Dash (any flavor).
2. Spray with Pam liberally.
3. Saute chicken in pan, brown on both sides (add garlic or onion, if desired).
4. When chicken is almost fully cooked add 2 tablespoons of light balsamic vinaigrette to pan with chicken to enhance flavor.
5. One bag of fresh spinach, steam or saute with garlic, add salt and pepper to taste
6. Sweet Potato - baked: pierce potato with fork or knife then bake in 350 degree oven until tender; or microwave (preferred method): pierce with knife or fork, microwave in 5 to 10 minute increments until tender.

Recipe 2:
Black Bean Turkey Burgers

1. 1 package of ground turkey (93% lean)
2. 1 can of black beans (drained)
3. Mix ground turkey and black beans; add salt and pepper.
4. Refrigerate patties for ½ hour or longer to firm up patties (turkey patties may also be frozen for later use
5. Spray pan liberally with Pam and add small amount of Canola Oil; then heat pan.

6. Put turkey patties in pan and cook entirely through (burgers cannot be eaten medium or rare). If pan seems to be burning, add a little water.
7. You may put this on a whole wheat bun, Sara Lee whole wheat sandwich thin, or whole wheat english muffin.

Recipe 3:
Avocado, Tomato and Chickpea Salad with Grilled Chicken (or Shrimp)

1. Cut 2 small tomatoes in cubes.
2. Dice 1 whole avocado.
3. Drain 1 whole can of chick peas.
4. Mix all Ingredients together. Add 1 tablespoon of olive oil, and salt and pepper to taste. Optional: add juice of ½ lime.
5. Serve and eat immediately!

(You may add grilled chicken or grilled shrimp for more protein.)

Recipe 4:
Salmon with Yogurt Lemon Dill Sauce

(Serves 4)

4 fresh salmon filets (skinless) - 6 oz. each
½ cup plain Greek yogurt
1 tablespoon of dried dill weed
Juice from ½ of a lemon
Salt and pepper

1. Salt and pepper salmon to taste. Saute or bake salmon until center is pink (do not overcook).
2. While salmon is cooking, mix together Greek yogurt, dill, and juice from lemon (add a touch of Splenda if too tart).

3. When salmon is cooked, transfer to plate. Add lemon, dill, and yogurt mixture on top of salmon filet.
4. Serving suggestion - serve with your favorite vegetable or salad.

Recipe 5:
Easy Chicken Soup

1-32 ounce carton/can of Chicken Stock
1 whole Onion (Peel but leave whole)
2 Celery Stalks
2 Cups cooked sliced carrots
1 Bag of Fresh Baby Spinach
1 Cup diced firm Tofu
2 cups cooked chicken cubed or shredded
1 cup of quartered cherry tomatoes

In a large stock pot add chicken stock, whole onion, and celery stalks, bring to a boil and then lower to simmer until celery and onion are tender. Pull out celery and onion. Cut up one stalk of celery and a quarter cup of the onion and return to pot. Add carrots, spinach, tofu, chicken, and tomatoes.

Turn up heat slightly, and cook until spinach is fully wilted and tomatoes are soft.

Serve with a hearty salad

SNACK

Recipe 1:

Greek yogurt (Chobani or Dannon Light & Fit; make sure you find a yogurt with less than 12 grams of sugar). Mix in 2 tablespoons of organic ground flaxseed and top with Reddi-Whip.

Recipe 2:

Take 5 strawberries and a handful of blueberries.
Mix with ½ cup cottage cheese.

Recipe 3:

2 hardboiled eggs
2 teaspoons hummus
Remove yolks of the hardboiled eggs and fill them with hummus.

Recipe 4:
Turkey and Swiss Cheese Roll-ups

3-4 slices of roast turkey
3-4 slices of Swiss cheese

Put one slice of turkey atop one slice of Swiss.
Put mustard, hummus, or your condiment of choice.
Roll up and *mangia!*

Recipe 5
Pb and J and CC
(Peanut Butter and Jelly and Cottage Cheese)

1. 1 or 2 slices of Whole Grain or whole wheat bread, Thomas English muffin or flatbread
2. 1 Teaspoon or Tablespoon of Peanut Butter
3. 1 Teaspoon of Polaner or Smuckers Natural Jelly
4. 1 Tablespoon of Cottage Cheese

Spread Pb, jelly and cottage cheese on bread, flatbread, muffin, etc.

Enjoy with a glass of water or Almond milk

SMOOTHIES

Recipe 1:
Blueberry Breakfast Smoothie

½ cup of blueberries
1 scoop of protein powder
½ cup of walnuts
Add 6-8 ounces of water and crushed ice.
Blend and enjoy!

Recipe 2:
Cereal Smoothie

½ cup of Cheerios, or Fiber One Cereal
6 oz. of almond milk
1 scoop of whey protein powder
1 tablespoon of peanut butter
Add crushed ice and blend.

Recipe 3:
Yogurt Almond Smoothie

1 cup of yogurt (plain preferred)
8 oz. of almond milk
½ cup of almonds
1 scoop of whey protein powder
Add crushed ice and blend.

Recipe 4:
PB and Whey Smoothie

1 tablespoon of peanut butter

1 scoop of whey protein powder
8 ounces of almond milk
Add crushed ice and blend.
Top with Reddi Whip.

Recipe 5:
Flax and Walnut Smoothie

1 tablespoon of ground flax
¼ cup of chopped walnuts
1 scoop of whey protein
1 cup of water, or almond or any kind of milk
Add crushed ice and blend.

Printed in the United States
By Bookmasters